Crossword Nurse

Puzzles and cartoons for nurses

Crossword Nurse

Crossword Nurse
Copyright © 2017 by Chris Hendricks
Art and illustrations by Kiana Hendricks

ISBN-10: 0-692-90375-5
ISBN-13: 978-0-692-90375-9

Preface

As a professional nurse educator I am always looking for better ways of learning. In this search I have discovered gamification, which is applying game elements to learning. Games are fun as we all know, but how does that lead to better learning?

One of the most effective ways to reinforce learning is through quizzes and tests. This is because you must recall information you have previously learned. Every time you recall information it is reinforced. Material that you recall all the time, let's say the dose of morphine, becomes second nature. Information that is never recalled is usually lost over time.

A crossword puzzle is a form of a test or quiz, but in a fun way. Professional nurses will get a kick out of testing their knowledge and practice. Student nurses will especially benefit. If you don't know the answer, it will point towards what to study. The puzzles reflect a professional level of knowledge.

Anyone who has served in triage will be able to relate to Triage Tales. Each and every one of these is rooted in reality! More than one of these episodes is taken almost verbatim from an encounter that a coworker or I have experienced. You really can't make this stuff up! I hope you enjoy the book, and maybe learn something along the way.

Chris Hendricks RN, MSN, CEN, CFN

—

This page left intentionally blank.

Contents

Crossword Puzzles

Crossword Solutions

Word Searches

Triage Tales

Graphic teaching

Nursing theory and ethics

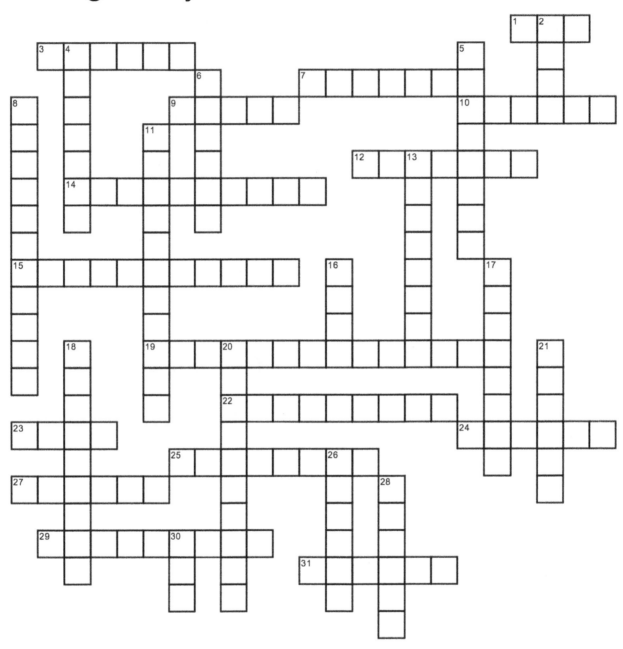

Across

1 Nurse Practice ____

3 Effort to manage stress

7 Sense of right and wrong

9 Humanbecoming- Rosemarie _____

10 Unitary model- Martha _____

12 See 16 down

14 Considers the right action, not the outcome

15 First nursing theorist

19 Do no harm

22 Ends justify the means

23 Goal Attainment model- Imogene ____

24 Moral composant of nursing

25 Control over self destiny

27 From Novice to Expert

29 14 Activities for Client Assistance- Virginia _____

31 Betty N_____ Systems model

Down

2 See 16 down

4 Nursing Process- Ida _____

5 Truth telling

6 Human Caring Science- Jean _____

8 13 Canons

11 Desire to do good

13 Notes on Nursing

16 Dorothea Orem model (3 wds. with 2 down and 12 across)

17 Being faithful

18 Transcultural- Madeline _____

20 Theory about a theory

21 Conservation model- Myra _____

26 Maternal Role attainment- Ramona _____

28 Health as Expanding Consciousness- Margaret _____

30 Adaptation model- Sister Calista ____

Play this puzzle for free online at;
https://crosswordhobbyist.com/300290
Password: supernurse

Watch the YouTube video to help study for this;
https://youtu.be/RDKpriwOEms

Crossword Nurse

Anatomy basics; regions and directions

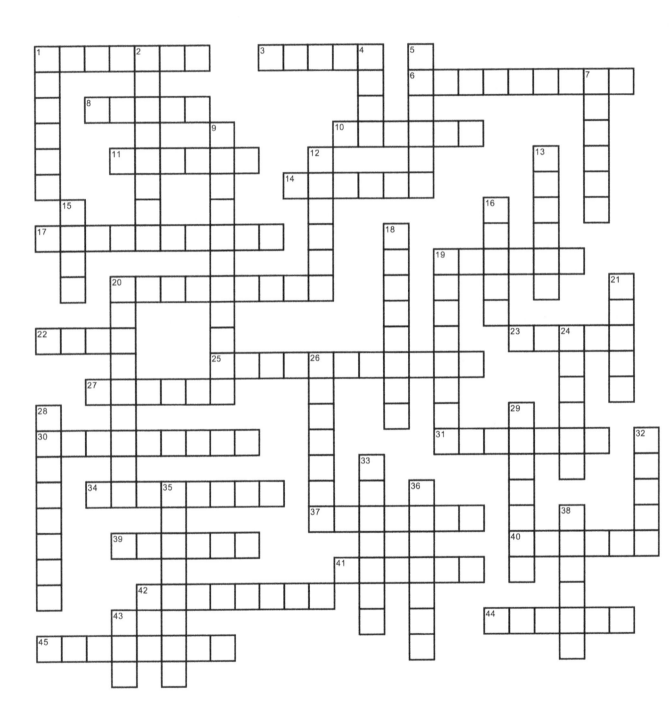

Across

1 Plane that divides front and back

3 Pubic

6 Back of elbow

8 Face down

10 Ankle

11 Great toe

14 Coccyx

17 Plane that divides top and bottom

19 Thumb

20 Back of knee

22 Lower leg

23 Thigh

25 Front of elbow

27 Chin

30 Belly button

31 Away from the longitudinal axis

34 Upper arm

37 Side lying

39 Face up

40 Armpit

41 Sole of foot

42 Separates left from right

44 Away from an attached base

45 Below

Down

1 Face

2 Chest

4 Calf

5 Back

7 Eye

9 Close to the surface

12 Wrist

13 Groin

15 Mouth

16 Palm

18 Front

19 Toward an attached base

20 Behind

21 Ear

24 Towards the longitudinal axis

26 Section of the skull

28 Above

29 Belly side

32 Cheek

33 Kneecap

35 The head

36 Skull

38 Fingers

43 Foot

Play this puzzle for free online at;
https://crosswordhobbyist.com/299032
Password: supernurse

Crossword Nurse

Nursing theory and ethics

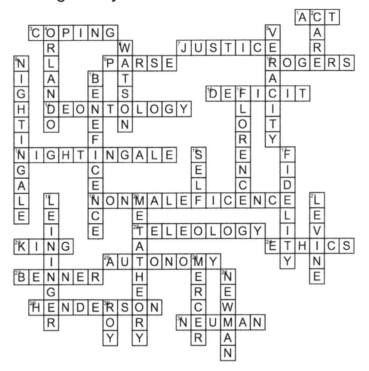

Anatomy basics; regions and directions

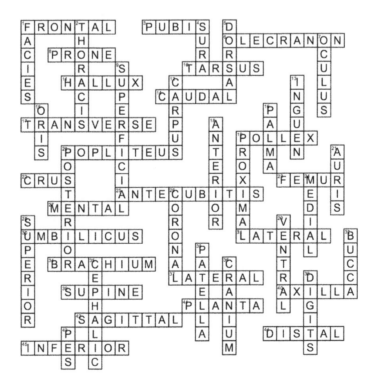

Crossword Nurse

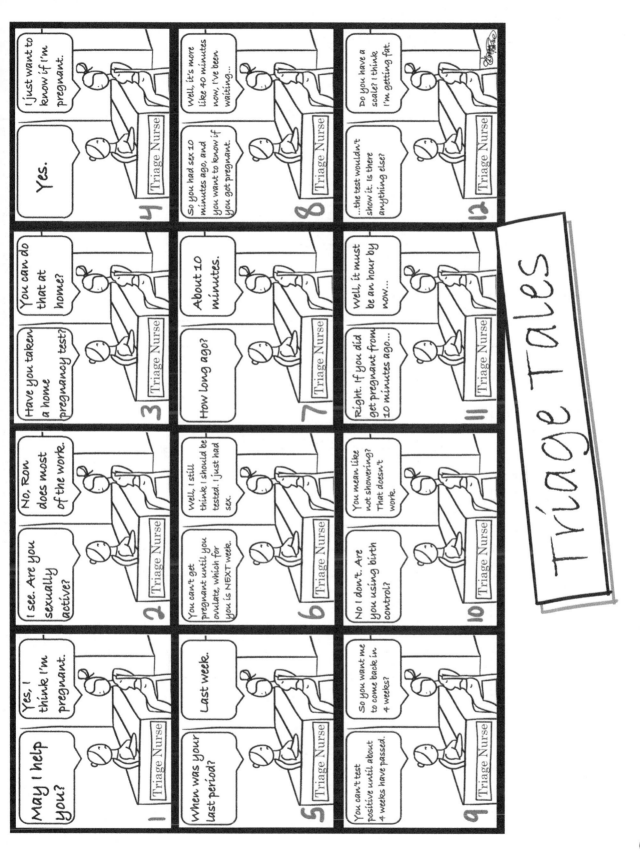

Triage Tales

Crossword Nurse

Pharmacology; Principles, administration

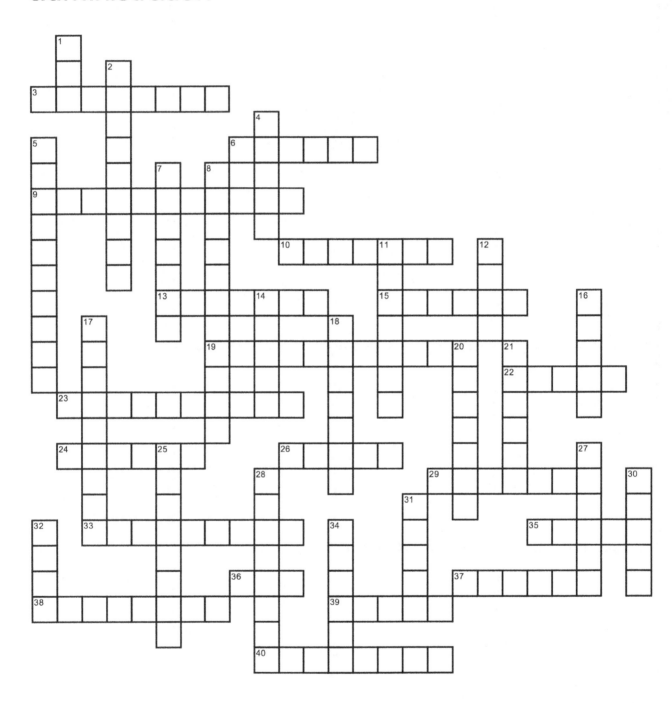

Across

3 Taken into the body

6 Lowest drug level

9 Hurts fetus

10 Remove from the body

13 Stimulates a receptor

15 With 39 across

19 Into the dermis

22 Preventable adverse medication event

23 Absorbed outside the GI tract

24 See 30 down

26 Time required for a drug to have an effect

29 Type of transport that requires no energy

33 When effect is greater than number of drugs

35 IM (with 28 down)

36 Under the tongue (with 20 down)

37 In the cheek

38 Movement of drug within body

39 Into the subarachnoid space (with 15 across)

40 Where the drug exerts effect

Down

1 SC (with 17 down)

2 When the body gets used to the drug

4 See 16 down

5 Block a receptor

7 Administered on the skin

8 Changed into excreted form

11 Absorbed by the GI tract

12 PO

14 IV (with 21 down)

16 Barrier that protects the brain (2 wds. with 4 down)

17 See 1 down

18 Undesired effect

20 See 36 across

21 See 14 down

25 Histamine release

27 PR

28 See 35 across

30 Med patch (with 24 across)

31 Organ that first pass refers to

32 Highest drug level

34 Type of transport that requires energy

Play this puzzle for free online at;
https://crosswordhobbyist.com/199913
Password: supernurse

Crossword Nurse

Cardiovascular drugs

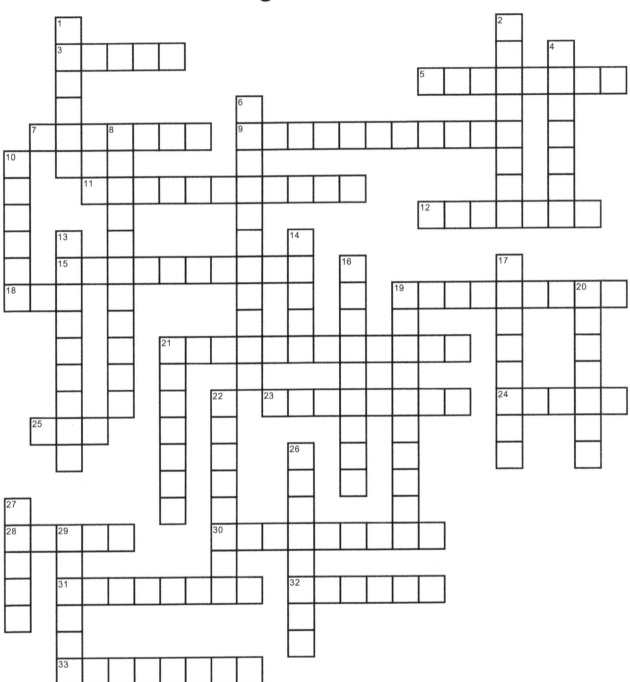

Across

3 Receptor in peripheral vasculature

5 How to reverse heparin (2 wds.)

7 Nifedipine is a(n) _____ channel blocker

9 Powerful alpha agonist for CPR

11 Adverse effect from too much beta blocker

12 Class of anti-lipid drugs

15 Type of drug that increases conduction in the heart

18 Captopril is a(n) _____ inhibitor

19 Nitro reduces _____

21 ACE Inhibitors are for _____

23 Polymorphic VTach

24 First choice for angina

25 Lab elevated in CHF

28 Prototype loop diuretic for acute CHF

30 Calcium channel blocker for Afib

31 Rescue drug for cardiogenic shock

32 What is the "O" in MONA

33 The "M" in MONA

Down

1 Most angiotensin II blockers end in _____

2 Plavix is an anti-_____

4 Prototype cardiac glycoside

6 Too much can cause low heart rate (2wds.)

8 Type that increases heart rate

10 Used for erectile dysfunction

13 May cause transient asystole

14 Location of Beta 1 receptors

16 Used for alcoholic torsades

17 Lab marker for acute MI

19 First choice for VFib

20 Antiplatelet used for MI

21 Prototype thrombin inhibitor

22 Low vitamin K diet

26 Type that increases pumping action of the heart

27 Terazosin is a(n) _____ blocker

29 Lidocaine is a(n) _____ channel blocker

Play this puzzle for free online at;
https://crosswordhobbyist.com/300320
Password: supernurse

Crossword Nurse

The Mechanics of CHF

CHF can be a difficult concept for students to grasp. This illustration will:

- explain CHF
- what it is
- how it works
- differentiate L vs. R heart failure
- how to treat it

<u>Let's say this is the heart at rest.</u>

1. During diastole, or between beats, the heart passively fills with blood, propelled by the diastolic blood pressure.

3. To complete systole, the ventricles contract. The amount they contract is the ejection fraction.

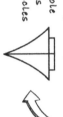

2. At the start of systole the atria contract. This "plumps" up the ventricles (see Starling's Law).

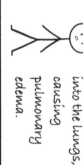

4. Notice how the ventricles are both the same size. They pump the same amount of blood. When there is an imbalance, and one ventricle can't pump equally to the other, it results in CHF.

Causes & Treatment

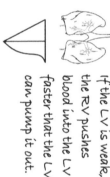

If the LV is weak, the RV pushes blood into the LV faster that the LV can pump it out.

Fluid will back up into the lungs, causing pulmonary edema.

If the RV is weak, the LV pushes blood into the RV faster that the RV can pump it out.

Fluid will back up into the body, causing peripheral edema.

-Chronic HTN
- ○Reduce afterload with nitrates, diuretics
- ○Block sympathetic tone with beta or alpha blockers
- ○ACE inhibitors do both of above

-Cardiomyopathy
- ○Stiff muscle mass inhibits normal beating
- ○Improve pumping action with digoxin
- ○May ultimately need transplant or VAD

-Acute MI
- ○Manage with MONA, cath lab, CABG
- ○Support pumping action with inotrope

-Valvular disease
- ○Percutaneous valvuloplasty, surgery

11

Fluids

```
Z B V C A F R G K P B R E A S T M I L K
L N B T S P N Y L Y H V R C N U H A F D
R G U V A F A K O M L K Q Z K V G I M Y
S P T P H L E M C V K O T X J K T N Y K
T L J I C A R S H A I W B J N P S T S H
F E J E H Z I M I G N B I L E Z P R E D
U U R Q Y G A E A I T Y T A S V U A R Z
C R D A M I U G V N E H C Q O I T C U E
S A Z I E T R M W A R K O U S T U E M X
P L S S A O J A T L S S L E A R M L H T
U P Y N N R P U K N T E O O N E A L M R
S L B M H S R A W M I R S U G O S L B A
T A P K P L Y H E J T O T S U U P U N C
E S Q U Z H B N E H I U R Z I S I L M E
A M I B R N R L O A A S U W N Z R A U L
R A F R U E O R O V L B M N E Q A R C L
S R P V R R L N W O I O M T O C T H U U
V O M I T T I E X W D A W N U H E U S L
K S A L I V A N N J H H L H S F H E V A
S R M H Z O D Q E T S E M E N Q O M O R
```

WORD LIST:

AQUEOUS
ASPIRATE
BILE
BLOOD
BREASTMILK
CHYME
COLOSTRUM
CSF
DIARRHEA

EXTRACELLULAR
INTERSTITIAL
INTRACELLLULAR
LOCHIA
LYMPH
MUCUS
PHLEM
PLASMA
PLEURAL

PURELENT
PUS
RHUEM
SALIVA
SANGUINEOUS
SEMEN
SEROUS
SERUM
SMEGMA

SPUTUM
SYNOVIAL
TEARS
URINE
VAGINAL
VITREOUS
VOMIT

You can find the solution for this puzzle at;
   https://mywordsearch.com/149874
   Password: supernurse

Crossword Nurse

Pharmacology; Principles, administration

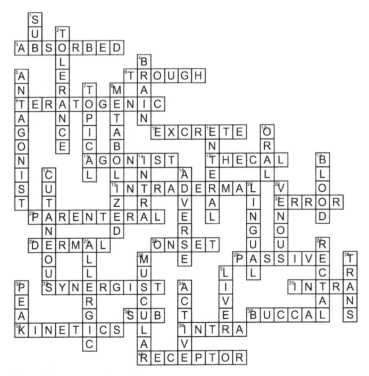

Cardiovascular drugs

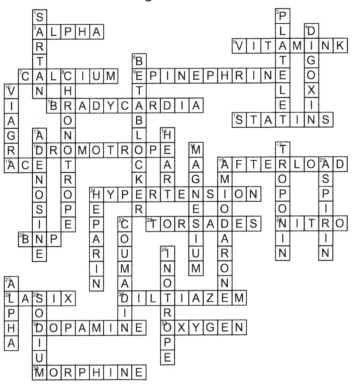

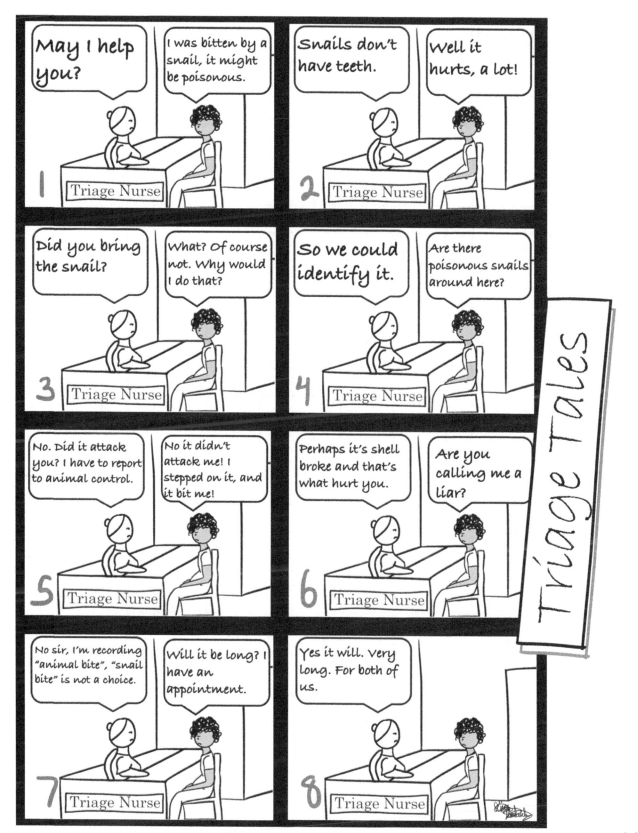

Crossword Nurse

Heart Attack

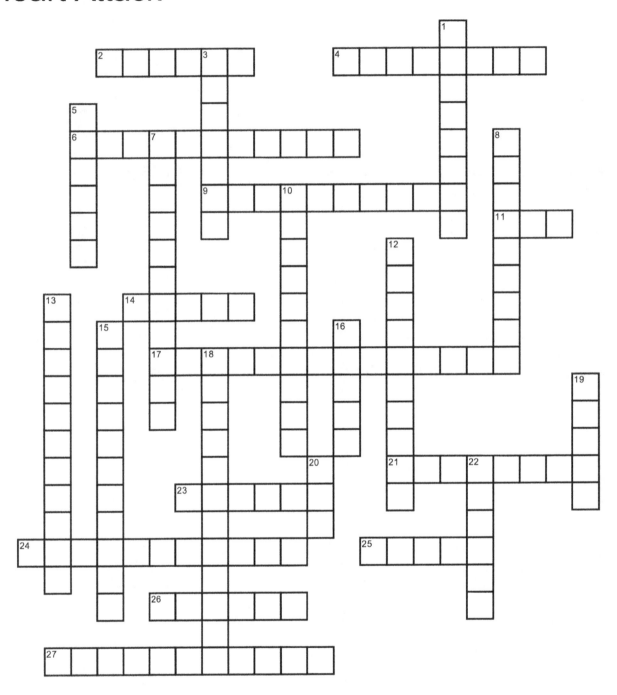

Across

2 Type of irregular, narrow tachycardia (with 18 down).

4 What lab test confirms MI?

6 Disorganized rhythm, no pulse (with 18 down).

9 See 12 down.

11 Responsive to Adenosine (abbr.)

14 What structure does papillary muscle rupture affect?

17 What "shocking" is called.

21 The term for flatline.

23 This substance, which when ruptures, can trigger an MI.

24 What do they perform in the cath lab?

25 What is the "N" in MONA? (abbr.)

26 Ratio of chest compressions to respirations; _____ to two.

27 Cardiogenic shock causes _____.

Down

1 What powerful pressor is given for cardiogenic shock?

3 What anti-platelet is proven to reduce mortality?

5 What structure pauses the heart beat to allow "atrial kick"? (2 wds.)

7 Too fast

8 Classic symptom of heart attack (2 wds.)

10 Calcium-sodium channel blocker used for arrhythmias.

12 Medical term for heart attack (with 9 across).

13 What is the first-line drug in CPR?

15 What sign on the 12 lead shows MI? (2 wds.)

16 What rhythm allows only some impulses to trigger a heart beat?

18 See 2 across, or 6 across.

19 Device used for symptomatic bradycardia (abbr.)

20 Auto shock device (abbr.)

22 What structure generates the heart beat? (abbr.)

Play this puzzle for free online at;
https://crosswordhobbyist.com/306284
Password: supernurse

Crossword Nurse

Nursing shift

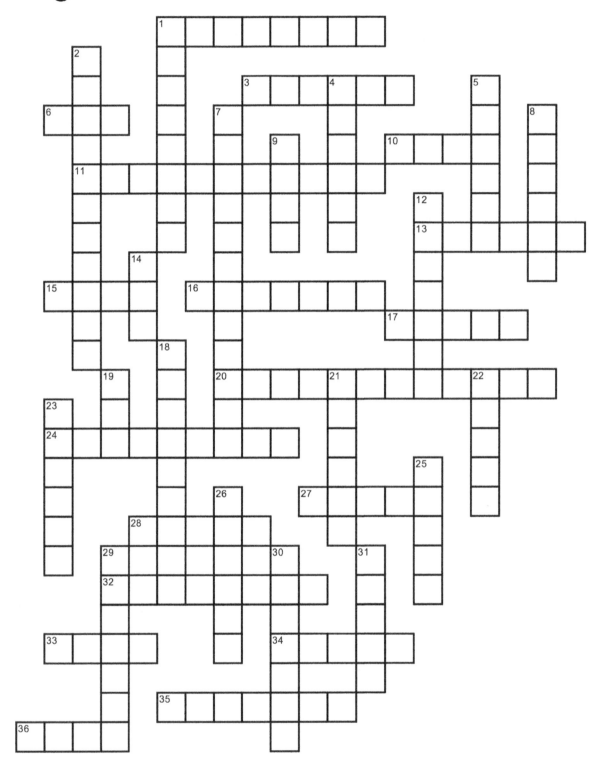

Across

1 What you use for emergencies (2 wds. with 4 down)

3 My patient is having a CVA (2 wds. with 22 down)

6 Common pediatric respiratory illness

10 What gravity can cause (2 wds. with 33 across)

11 Bad IV

13 Type of nurse on contract

15 Slang for soiled patient (2 wds. with 27 across)

16 My patient is having an MI (2 wds. with 22 down)

17 Type of mini seizure

20 Type of suction

24 What you fill out after med error (2 wds. with 21 down)

27 See 15 across

28 See 9 down

32 _____ fixation

33 See 10 across

34 Privacy act

35 _____ precautions

36 Code for arrest

Down

1 Conscious _____

2 Who you call if your patient is wheezing (2 wds. with 18 down)

4 See 1 across

5 See 23 down

7 See 12 down

8 Specialist who performs swallow screen (2 wds. with 18 down)

9 Patient signaling device (2 wds. with 28 across)

12 What the survey wants (2 wds. with 7 down)

14 Trach and ____

18 See 2 down or 8 down

19 Wound ___

21 What you get at start of shift

22 See 16 across or 3 across

23 IV fluid (2 wds. with 5 down)

25 Treatment for constipation

26 Head nurse

29 Preferred type of hand-off report

30 Where angioplasty is performed (2 wds. abbr.)

31 Works in multiple departments

Play this puzzle for free online at;
https://crosswordhobbyist.com/318745
Password: supernurse

Crossword Nurse

Heart Attack

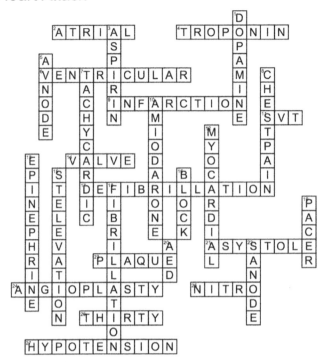

Nursing shift

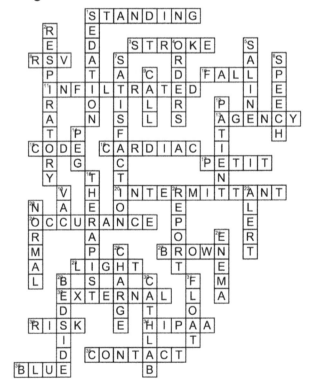

Crossword Nurse

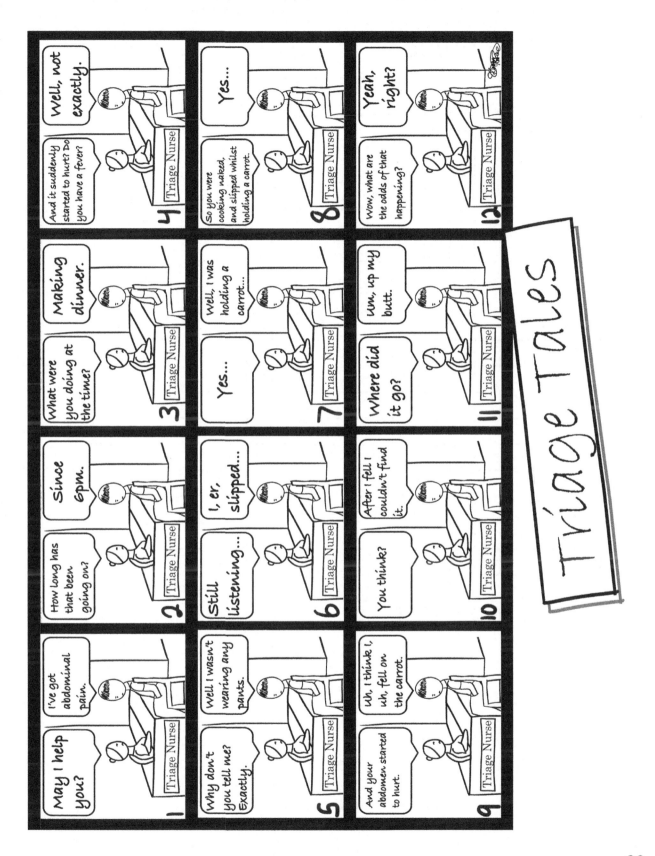

Crossword Nurse

Respiratory drugs

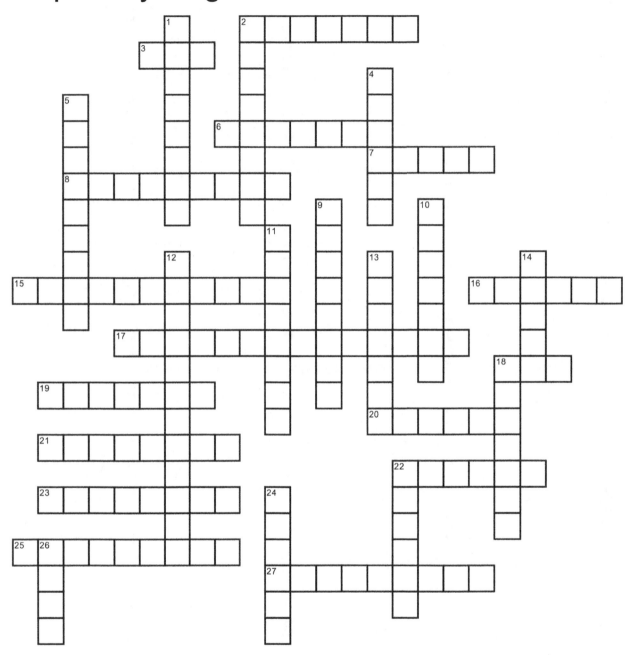

Across

2 What substance reacts to a specific antibody?

3 Common adverse effect to Atrovent (With 14 down)

6 What structure in the airway does not contract nor dilate?

7 Term for "barky" seal-like cough

8 What is the term for breathing fast?

15 What powerful bronchodilator can be given IM?

16 What is the term used for the drug combo Albuterol and Atrovent?

17 Opens the airways

18 Condition in which fluid backs up into the lungs. (abbr.)

19 Term to describe the sound mucus and fluid in the airways

20 What is the most important drug for any respiratory emergency?

21 What is a very effective way to measure the severity of asthma? (2 wds.)

22 What is the term for normal breathing?

23 What common stimulant should patients taking theophylline avoid?

25 Causes a "barrel" chest to develop

27 Prototype beta 2 agonist

Down

1 What is an inhaled anti-inflammatory used for prophylaxis?

2 What substance evokes an inflammatory response?

4 What device will increase the effectiveness of an inhaler?

5 The "P" in DTAP

9 Lower airway obstruction causes this sound

10 Upper airway obstruction causes _____.

11 What is the normal ratio of inhalation to exhalation? (3 wds.)

12 What is the prototype methylxanthine?

13 Receptor in the lungs (2 wds.)

14 See 3 across

18 What is a common infection that can result from chronic inhaled glucocorticoid use?

22 Lifesaving device carried by people allergic to bees

24 What is the drug combo Fluticasone and Salmeterol called?

26 What cells release histamine?

Play this puzzle for free online at;
https://crosswordhobbyist.com/302177
Password: supernurse

My hormones

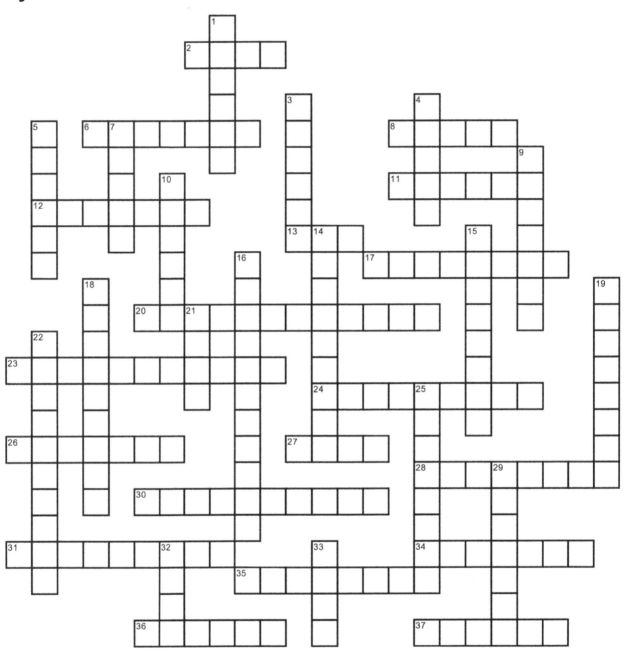

Across

2 Insulin is produced in the _____ cells.

6 See 21 down

8 Progesterone

11 Responsible for growth

12 TSH targets the _____.

13 Adrenal product, (abbr.)

17 Stimulates sperm maturation

20 Pituitary attached to _____

23 Thyroid neighbor

24 Also known at T4

26 Anti-diuretic hormone targets the _____.

27 Drug that reabsorbs water (with 15 down)

28 Thymus

30 Melanin in skin

31 Lives in sella turcica

34 Pancreas makes

35 Pancreas makes

36 Corticosteroids are produced in the adrenal _____.

37 See 32 down

Down

1 Released by fat cells

3 The thymus is key in the _____ system.

4 Estrogen

5 Testosterone

7 Organ that makes B natriuretic peptide

9 "Hunger" hormone

10 Organ source of Erythropoietin

14 Promotes milk production

15 See 27 across

16 Stimulates ovulation

18 Pineal gland makes _____

19 Pancreatic alpha cells produce _____

21 Stimulates osteoslcasts (with 6 across)

22 Lowers blood calcium levels.

25 Released by breast feeding

29 Epinephrine is produced in the adrenal _____.

32 Too much growth hormone causes _____. (With 37 across)

33 Abbreviation for adrenocorticotropic hormone

Play this puzzle for free online at;
https://crosswordhobbyist.com/296580
Password: supernurse

Crossword Nurse

Respiratory drugs

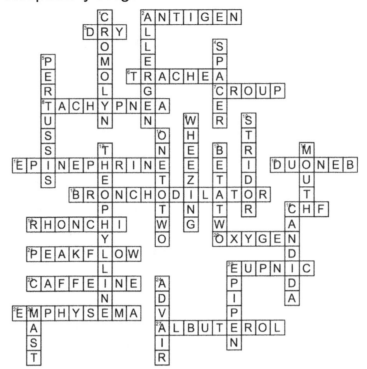

My hormones

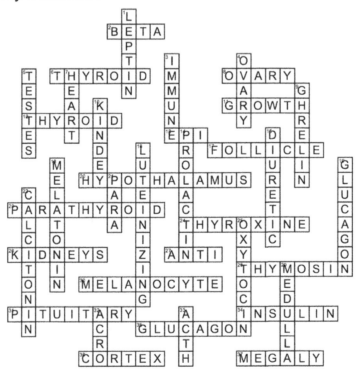

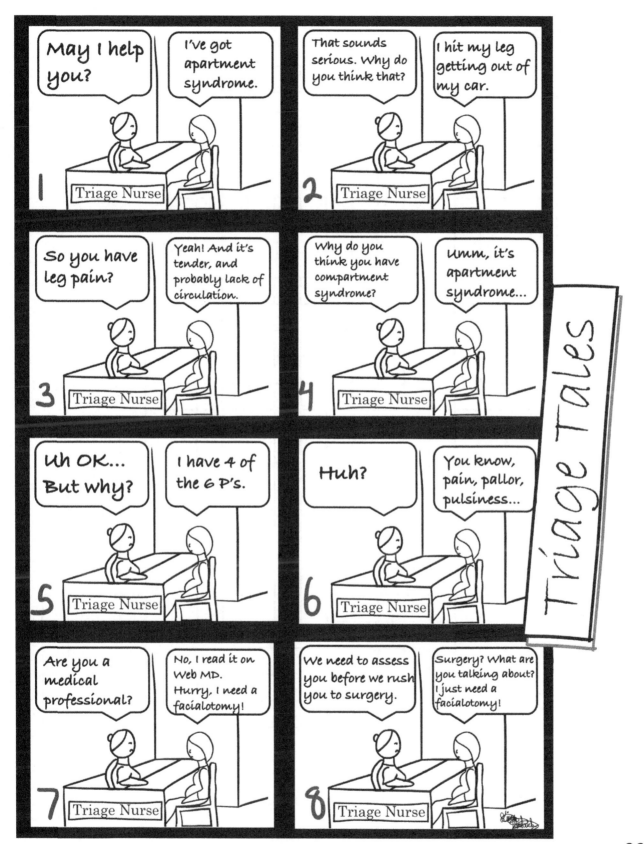

Crossword Nurse

Trauma

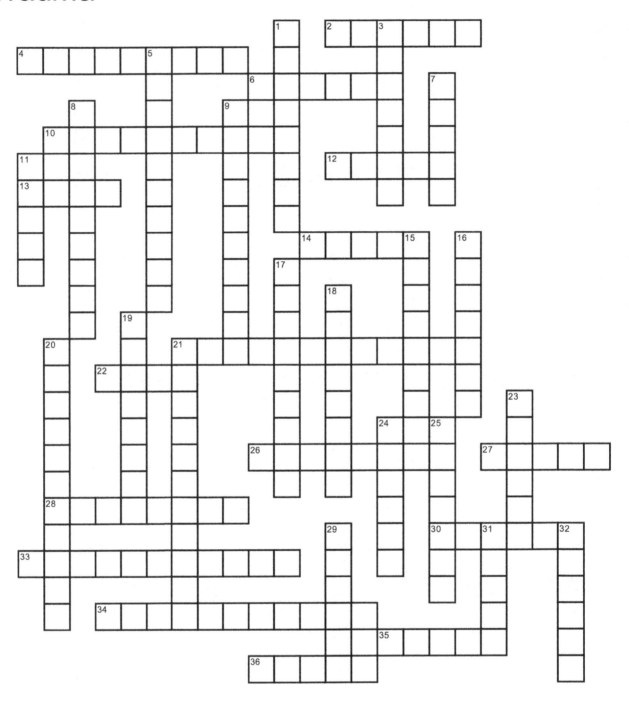

Across

2 See 11 down

4 Traumatic separation of the placenta and uterine wall.

6 Contusion

10 Tear in the skin

12 Causes penetrating trauma

13 Drowning victims often have _____ (with 3 down).

14 Cold injury (with 22 across)

21 Type of shock from excessive bleeding

22 See 14 across

26 Collection of blood in tissues

27 This triad shows; JVD, muffled heart tones, and hypotension.

28 Body part torn away but still attached

30 System of classifying facial fractures

33 When a joint is disrupted

34 System for estimating burned body surface area (3 wds.)

35 See 25 down

36 Type of trauma suffered in frontal car crash

Down

1 Pertaining to evidence.

3 See 13 across

5 Treatment for life threatening bleeding from an extremity

7 Large organ most often injured in blunt trauma

8 Term for fluid or blood in epicardial space

9 Study of how energy in motion impacts the body

11 Procedure to open the chest (with 2 across)

15 Type of pneumothorax that is the most life threatening

16 Blood collection in the anterior eye

17 Type of skull fracture likely from a blow from a hammer

18 Bleeding on the surface of the brain

19 Bleeding between the skull and the dura mater

20 Type of trauma suffered from a stabbing

21 Posturing seen after brain injury, arms pulled towards the core

23 Free air in the chest (with 32 down)

24 Type of organ most likely to be injured from pressure wave like an explosion

25 Clear fluid from an ear probably means this type of fracture. (With 35 across)

29 Organ in the left abdomen often injured in blunt trauma

31 Term for multiple ribs fractured in multiple places

32 See 23 down

Play this puzzle for free online at;
https://crosswordhobbyist.com/300466
Password: supernurse

Crossword Nurse

I've got a fever.

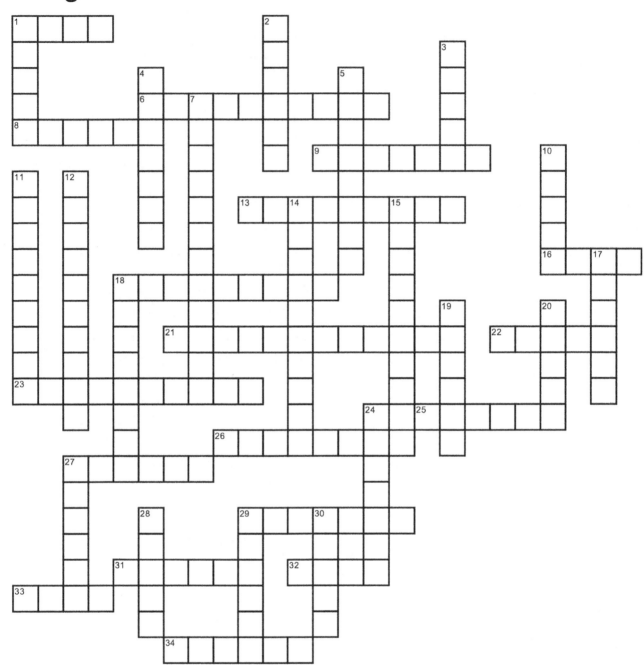

Across

1 First identified drug resistant strain (abbr.).

6 Immunization generates _____.

8 Term for overwhelming infection.

9 Rubeola

13 Increased blood flow is called _____.

16 Will kill a bacteria (with 31 across)

18 Treats herpes

21 Septic shock is also referred to as _____ shock.

22 See 20 down

23 Source of Lyme disease.

25 H2 antagonist

26 Adult varicella

27 Mediates cell immunity

29 Pathogen introduced to provoke immune response.

31 See 16 across

32 When sepsis gets worse. (abbr.)

33 Carries an infectious agent.

34 Anti-nausea med.

Down

1 Paratitis

2 Type of fluid that weeps from non-infected wound.

3 Cells that fight infection. (With 20 down and 22 across).

4 Breastfeeding gives us _____ immunity.

5 H1 antagonist

7 Can stain tooth enamel

10 Hemorrhagic fever

11 Infection in the liver.

12 Drug of choice for MRSA.

14 Prototype antibiotic

15 Vector for malaria

17 First lymphoid organ of the GI tract.

18 TB requires _____ precautions.

19 First generation broad spectrum cephalosporin.

20 See 3 down

24 Causes tetony

27 Immune organ shrinks markedly with aging.

28 Source of mad cow disease.

29 Organism that carries infection between different animals.

30 Common vancomycin secondary infection (abbr.).

Play this puzzle for free online at;
https://crosswordhobbyist.com/314918
Password: supernurse

Crossword Nurse

Trauma

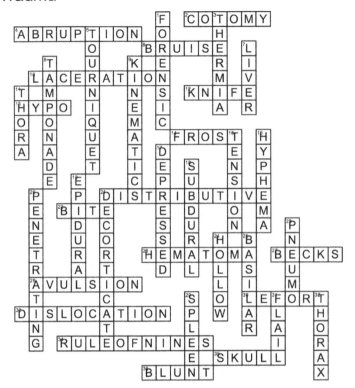

I've got a fever.

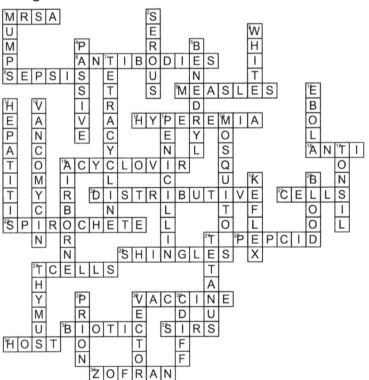

Crossword Nurse

Antibiotics and friends

```
R F Q D A C A E G N N H R U H Y O A T Y X X R R O E P Z C T
W M L Y C Y L J M E I T W Q M E I A Z A V O E B C F F Z V V
S U E U N N P E Q X Q P U F B M K J L C E F T I N H N A Z G
L Y C T C Z G Y O H A F L A G Y L G E N T A M I C I N N O K
N J M T R O Z F G C S U L P H A Z I O N D L E V T A V A O Q
I Y A M E O N S H J I D M D F A M P I C I L L I N Q A M Q X
Q E C Q D T N A N R G N F U Z E O N N P M I E I A R N I M S
P U R S I Y R I Z V J W E Z M P K P A D L A O C M P C V I A
T U O P P J P A D O Y A M A N T A D I N E C N H O T O I O D
U P D Q O U S O C A L T L F X P O X T I R O B L X D M R A K
A S A X S M J W Q Y Z E R W W J S C M D J G F O I T Y Q T J
L D N U Y S Y Q C U C O U F D Z E E L R S K A R C P C T Y E
P F T F T U C V K G R L L S T N L T J I Z K R O I L I V P F
T R I U C D S P P W X T I E I F T R D B W R D Q L K N T C D
J M N P L C B R P I U G V N Y V A I M O V X K U L I U Z P O
N R Y R I U U V T T I X C G E R M A C V F M X O I C E X E X
T I S J N A Z D I F L U C A N M I X N I R P P N N E R C N Y
J U T F D B E W G D F R C L I O V O N R I V J E A I Y K I C
T B A O A H B I A X I N I V P T I N V I A A G C Y N T Q C Y
F L T U M P N L I X N N P E K A R E D N A L Y H O G H I I C
S R I B Y A R E M S H U R P M M E L Y V J O X U C H R J L L
A I N Q C S O P I Z M D O K R I R C Z H S P V Z X F O Z L I
N F B X I P C Q P P L E F C E F I P I M E R M V I E M I I N
C A Z L N K E Q E U E P O H T L C E F A Z O L I N H Y T N E
E M Y W C V P S N O V F X E R U F B W F S I H Y B J C H I L
F P V X K J H H E I Q B A Q O F T S Y Y A C Y C O V I R B C
A I O N X A I A M C U U C U V Y R D R Y E A H Y U I N O L I
X N X K Z A N L G E I J I B I D U D E S W C S G P E R M I P
Q R I B I V I R I N N Y N Q R S E G H H Z I S C T K T A N R
E I S O N I A Z I D R L Y J Z Z A O J A P D E U T X B X I O
```

WORD LIST:

ACYCIOVIR	CIPRO	IMIPENEM	RIFAMPIN
AMANTADINE	CIPROFIOXACIN	ISONIAZID	ROCEPHIN
AMOXICILLIN	CLEOCIN	LEVAQUIN	SULPHA
AMPICILLIN	CLINDAMYCIN	MACRODANTIN	TAMIFLU
ANCEF	DIFLUCAN	METRONIDAZOLE	TETRACYCLINE
BIAXIN	DOXYCYCLINE	NYSTATIN	VALOPROICACID
CEFAZOLIN	ERYTHROMYCIN	OSELTAMIVIR	VANCOMYCIN
CEFIPIME	FLAGYL	PENICILLIN	ZANAMIVIR
CEFTIN	FLUCONAZOLE	RETROVIR	ZITHROMAX
CETRIAXONE	FUZEON	RIBIVIRIN	ZYVOX
CHLOROQUONE	GENTAMICIN	RIBOVIRIN	

Crossword Nurse

Party on!

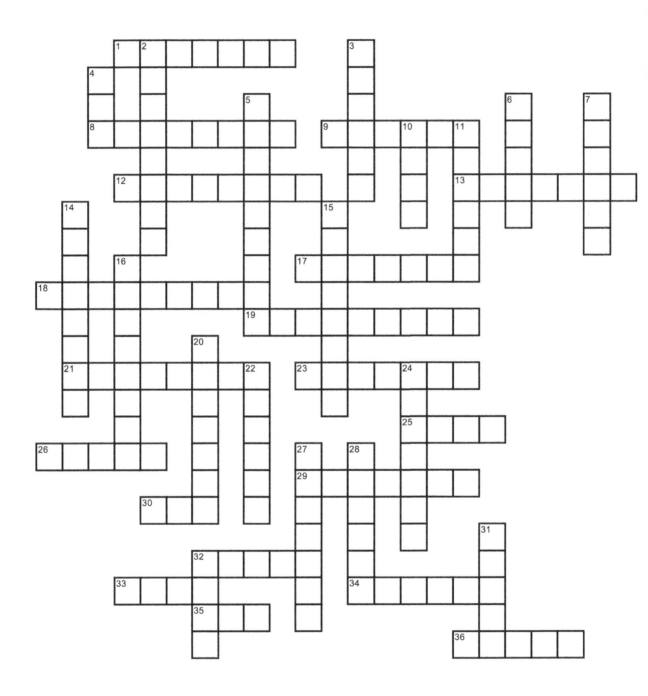

Across

1 Chemical name of alcohol

8 See 19 across

9 Antagonizes opioids

12 Active drug in cigarettes.

13 See 6 down

17 Life threatening complication of alcohol withdrawal

18 Benzodiazepine antagonist

19 Black drink for OD (2 wds. with 8 across)

21 Abused by body builders

23 A common cause of nystagmus

25 Sign of cocaine use (3 wds. with 36 across and 33 across)

26 Most dangerous effect of narcotic OD

29 PO drug to treat ETOH withdrawal

30 Prototype hallucinogen

32 See 32 down

33 See 25 across

34 See 35 across

35 Test for drug use (2 wds. with 34 across)

36 See 25 across

Down

2 Compulsive behaviors shown by meth users

3 Pinpoint pupils are a sign of _____ use.

4 Active drug in marijuana

5 Can cause hyper-emesis syndrome

6 Dangerous adverse effect of Ecstasy (with 13 across)

7 Compulsive user of a drug

10 Scale to measure degree of withdrawal

11 What to use for GI irrigation (2 wds.)

14 Antidote for acetaminophen overdose

15 Street name for Ketamine (2 wds.)

16 Active drug in coffee

20 Stimulants cause _____ pupils.

22 Drinking too much water causes low _____.

24 Inhaling gas is called _____.

27 Most abused drug

28 Unsanitary injections can cause _____.

31 Drinking a large amount at one time.

32 Ugly cosmetic effect of meth (2 wds. with 32 across).

Play this puzzle for free online at;
https://crosswordhobbyist.com/314932
Password: supernurse

34

Crossword Nurse

Stroke

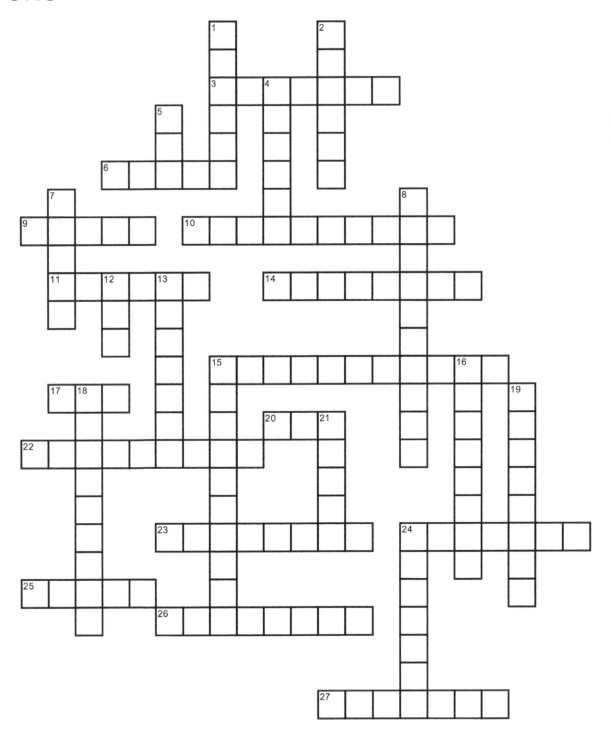

Crossword Nurse

Across

3 All acute stroke victims need a _____ screen.

6 Organ affected by stroke

9 With 11 across

10 Slurred speech

11 Common stoke symptom (2 wds. with 9 across)

14 Area of brain that can cause receptive aphasia

15 Worst kind of stroke

17 Clot buster (abbr.)

20 Stroke risk factor (abbr.)

22 Difficulty swallowing

23 Common cause of hemorrhagic stroke

24 Intravascular intervention

25 Area of brain that can cause expressive aphasia

26 Symptom of hemorrhagic stroke

27 Unaware of one side

Down

1 Imaging for stroke (2 wds.)

2 Circle of _____

4 Can't walk straight

5 Mini stroke (abbr.)

7 Can't hold arm straight

8 Stroke scale that assesses facial droop, arm drift, and speech.

12 Abbreviation for stroke.

13 Can't think of the word

15 Can't move one side

16 Less severe of the two types of stroke.

18 Type of stoke that originates from vertebral arteries.

19 Risk of t-PA

21 _____ stroke scale (abbr.)

24 Type of nerve that controls eye movement.

Play this puzzle for free online at;
https://crosswordhobbyist.com/318716
Password: supernurse

Party on!

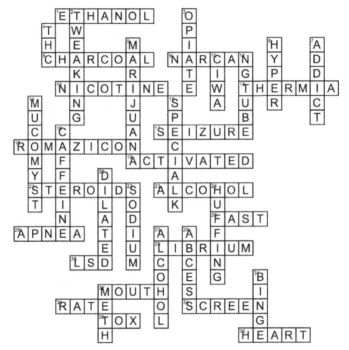

Stroke

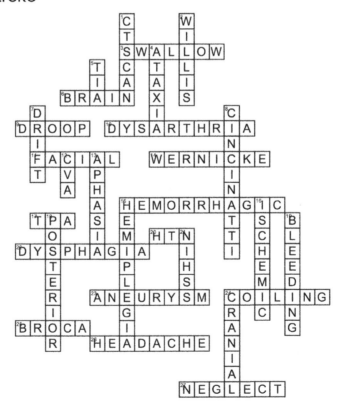

Crossword Nurse

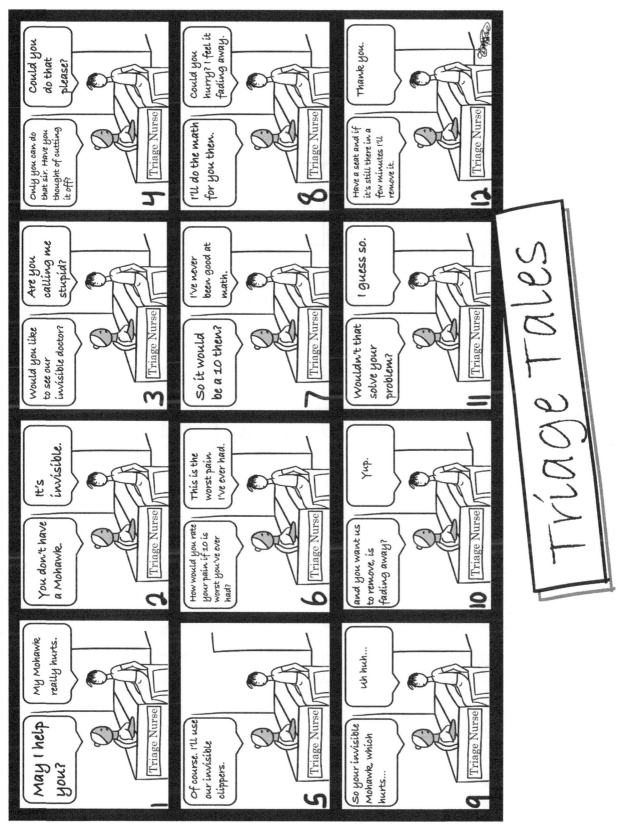

38

Crossword Nurse

Diabetes

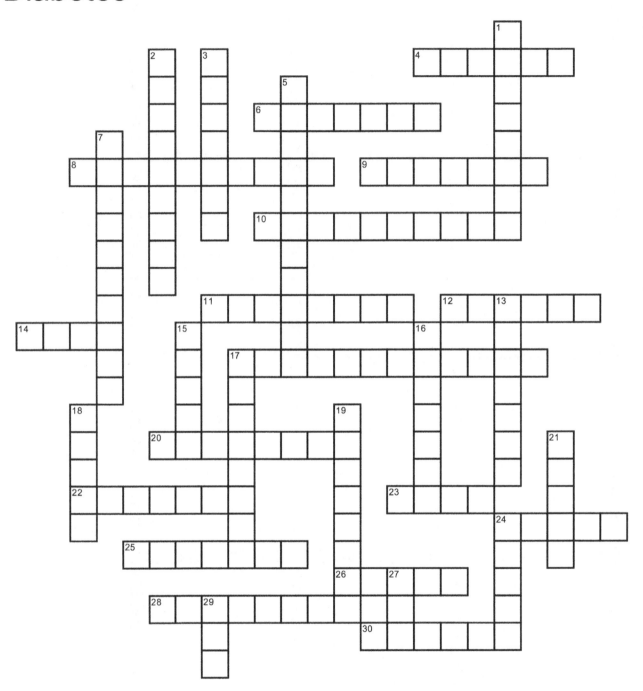

Across

4 See 24 across

6 Short acting insulin

8 See 17 across

9 See 15 down

10 Drinking too much water

11 IV drug for hypoglycemia

12 See 24 across

14 Instruction for glucose test

17 Blood test to show average blood sugar over time (2 wds. with 8 across)

20 Measure of how a food impacts blood sugar (2 wds. with 26 across)

22 Rapid insulin

23 Cells that make insulin

24 Instructions for mixing insulins (3 wds. with 4 across and 12 across)

25 Byproducts of fat metabolism

26 See 20 across

28 Organ that makes insulin

30 Long acting insulin

Down

1 Excessive urination

2 Prototype hyperglycemic drug

3 Medication for type I

5 ENT complication of diabetes

7 Numbness in feet

13 Lifestyle risk for diabetes

15 Reason for dialysis (2 wds. with 9 across)

16 Treatment for hypoglycemia

17 Rescue drug given IM

18 Cells that make glucagon

19 Metabolic disturbance in DKA

21 Major loss in DKA

24 Bad diet item (abbr.)

27 Hyperglycemic crisis (abbr.)

29 Cloudy insulin (abbr.)

Play this puzzle for free online at;
https://crosswordhobbyist.com/318733
Password: supernurse

Med-surg

```
A N E M I A S O R E S G Y K H M G T K X L F W L J D B E Y N
W P K F Y K K C R A C K L E S O Z R O F V E G K W M J A B A
T W E L V E L E A D E Q U T P E D A L A L V W H V R A M D S
D S F D D S D Q T C A C H E T I C L N W B E U X V I Y T Q O
N H D P H V N O R M A L G W W H F E B H H R C O U G H V C G
X V E N T R I C U L A R P B Y A R S C E V M R H O N C H I A
I N I T U B E B R A D Y C A R D I A V E C Y T E A D V T H S
Q C K W U C A T H E T E R W N K C O A Z Y O R D J Q N Q V T
D D S O R X D T K B U H P N P Z T Y T I A C A E F E X H W R
D W A U Z M P X V W V B O W E L I S U N N A C M Q X F E I I
V B L N T A C H Y C A R D I A X O Y W G O R H A S T I M N C
H T I D N L V I I N T E R N A L N I Y O T D T T E E N O F Y
Y C N V T S J F N I U H F O L E Y E M R I I R U R R F T L H
P C E A H Q Z H E M A T O C R I T J T M C A A Q O N A H A B
O M H C A S P I R A T I O N F G R U B A O L C G U A R O M Z
X K Q E Q N V J E S A N G U I N E O U S M B T K S L C R M N
I X P I E N E U G A T E L E C T E S I S U P I L W Z T A A F
C E K Z N S B L I Q U A R N P O S I N U S D O L N O I X T I
D I E P C F Y Z M D H G Y Z A Y B Y W H L K N N I I O A I B
I N D R F I I K E M B O L U S E F F U S I O N A A Z N W O R
Y F E B T I A L N P N E U M O T H O R A X P V G H D E N N I
A E H Q P U S L T J Y R Q E J Y M U C O S A S W M B E R S L
L C I K O H W Z U R M E K S F G R Z Q P R E S S U R E U Z L
X T S I S C H E M I A V K J R I D S P L I N T I N G A J L A
B I C T X F Y T Q F O T I N P S X M E Q B I H U N Y A F Y T
W O E J G A Y Q N Z S L I N G E W A P A M P F B O F O B B I
E N N C H E M I S T R Y E O Z L M N T I Y Z X B V U T I Q O
Q Q S G U T N W C I U K B B N E B X I I P D V H M G C M D N
L J E K T J N T H R O M B U S D D D X N O W E T T O D R Y A
Y D I T R A N S F U S I O N T H R U S H I N S X P M D X T Z
```

WORD LIST:

ANEMIA
ASPIRATION
ATELECTESIS
BOWEL
BRADYCARDIA
CACHETIC
CATHETER
CHEESY
CHEMISTRY
COUGH
CRACKLES
CVA
CYANOTIC
DEHISCENSE
DVT
EDEMA
EFFUSION

EMBOLUS
EXTERNAL
FEVER
FIBRILLATION
FIXATION
FOLEY
FRICTION
HEMATOCRIT
HEMOTHORAX
HYPOXIC
IMMOBILIZER
INFARCTION
INFECTION
INFILTRATION
INFLAMMATION
INTERNAL
ISCHEMIA

MUCOSA
MYOCARDIAL
NASOGASTRIC
NORMAL
PEDAL
PNEUMOTHORAX
PRESSURE
PUS
RALES
REGIMEN
RHONCHI
RUB
SALINE
SANGUINEOUS
SEROUS
SINUS
SLING

SORE
SPLINTING
TACHYCARDIA
TAMPONADE
THROMBUS
THRUSH
TIA
TRACH
TRACTION
TRANSFUSION
TUBE
TWELVELEAD
UTI
VENTRICULAR
WETTODRY
WHEEZING
WOUNDVAC

You can find the solution for this puzzle at;
https://mywordsearch.com/149857
Password: supernurse

Crossword Nurse

GI drugs

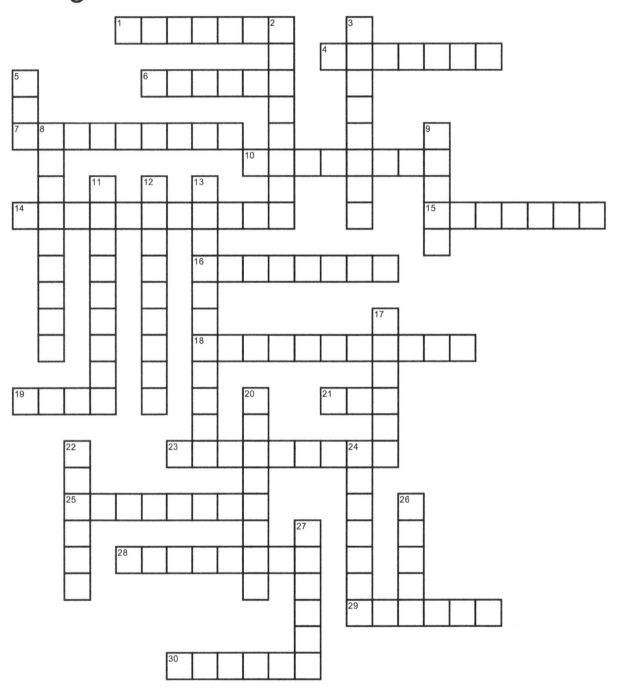

Across

1 Type of drug that fights acid

4 THC derived anti-nausea drug

6 Old-school vomit inducer

7 Hyper-osmotic laxative that reduces ammonia levels

10 Drug type that promotes elimination

14 Intestinal gas bubble reducer

15 Prototype H2 receptor antagonist

16 First proton pump inhibitor available IV

18 Probiotic

19 Suffix for H2 receptor antagonist

21 Prototype OTC antacid (abbr.)

23 Bulk forming laxative

25 Prototype proton pump inhibitor

28 Mucosal protectant, used for ulcers

29 Brand name Aluminum salt antacid

30 Serotonin blocker anti-nausea drug

Down

2 Stool softener

3 Cell that secretes acid

5 Type of acid in stomach (abbr.)

8 Drug that binds other drugs and toxins, used for oral OD (2 wds. with 20 down)

9 Brand name for bismuth subsalicylate (2 wds. with 17 down)

11 Antihistamine anti-nausea drug, good for dizziness

12 Anti-dopaminergic anti-nausea drug

13 Anticholinergic anti-nausea drug, used for seasickness

17 See 9 down

20 See 8 down

22 Newest generation H2 receptor antagonist

24 Anti-diarrheal that inhibits peristalsis

26 Common OTC stimulant laxative

27 Stomach enzyme that breaks down protein

Play this puzzle for free online at;
https://crosswordhobbyist.com/327519
Password: supernurse

Nervous system drugs

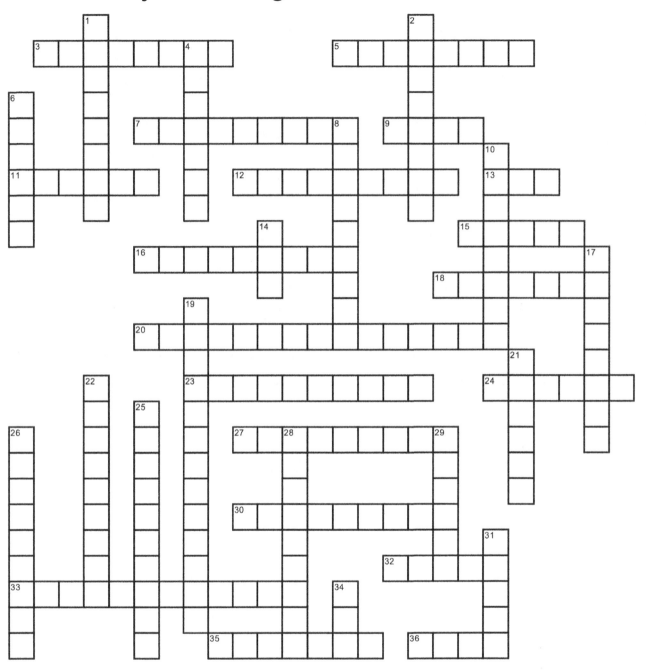

Across

3 Prototype opioid pain drug

5 Prototype anti-seizure drug

7 Dopamine replacing anti-Parkinson's drug (2 wds. with 17 down)

9 Street name for this pervasive illegal stimulant

11 Class of prototype pain drug

12 Drug of choice for treating opioid addiction

13 Test to record brain wave activity

15 Hallmark sign of Parkinson's

16 Commonly used sodium channel blocker, local anesthetic

18 Electoral storm in the brain

20 Prototype depolarizing agent

23 Anesthetic eye drops

24 Prototype anti-psychotic

27 Benzodiazepine antagonist

30 Original anti-depressant

32 Common anxiolytic anti-depressant

33 See 28 down

35 Serotonin antagonist used for treating migraines

36 Theory of pain transmission (2 wds. with 6 down)

Down

1 Milky white anesthetic

2 Widely consumed OTC stimulant

4 Laughing gas (2 wds. with 31 down)

6 See 36 across

8 Term for pain relieving drug

10 Street name is special K

14 Suffix for barbiturates

17 See 7 across

19 Most widely used OTC drug for pain

21 Prototype benzodiazepine

22 Key villain in opioid epidemic

25 GABA based anti-seizure drug

26 Natural endogenous pain killer

28 Life threatening adverse reaction to anesthesia (2 wds. with 35 across)

29 Prototype opioid antagonist

31 See 4 down

34 Suffix for inhaled anesthesia drugs

Play this puzzle for free online at;
https://crosswordhobbyist.com/328578
Password: supernurse

GI drugs

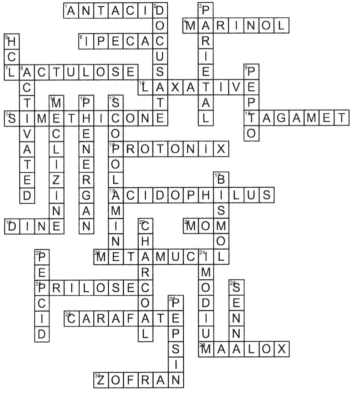

Nervous system drugs

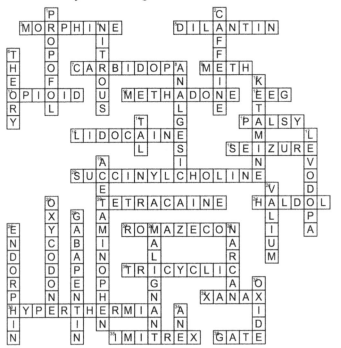

Crossword Nurse

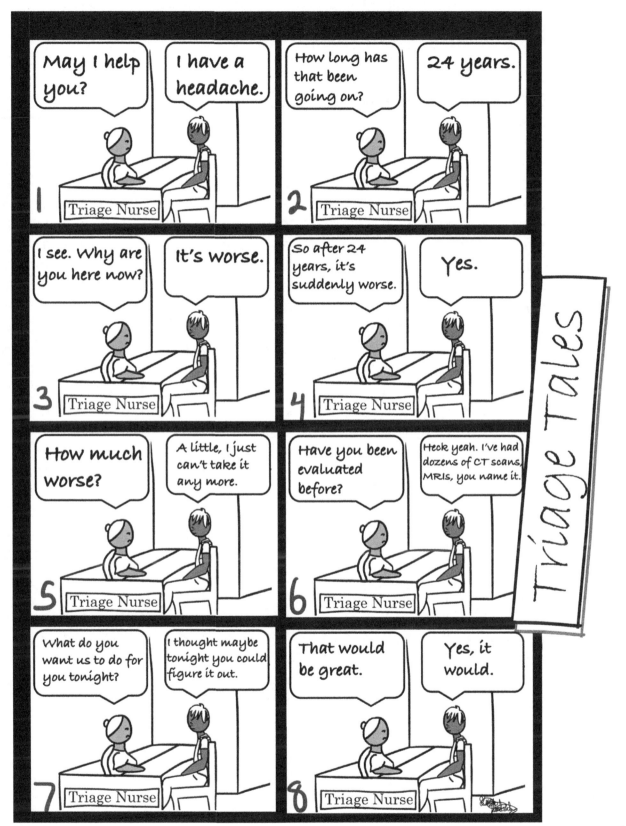

Crossword Nurse

Cath lab

```
L C W Y C E U J Q D F V Z T A C H Y C A R D I A I B S Z B N
A W E M B O L E C T O M Y H Y P E R A C U T E V V O T E O S
D B K P K T A A I N F E R I O R M I V T A C H J C N D B M T
W B P C J E Q T S S U P R E V E N T R I C U L A R R E M V N
J A C Q I C B G R E N P B V Y P V C Y F D M W E B C P S C X
M L K M G R A D A O C A T S Z F F M N A Y M J P V A R I S M
A L W Q M A C W N G P O E W R S W B A B E U A I B D E M E Z
T O R I W J V U P A A I N F A Z P N W H H F V N J P S T Q T
C O F U N A P F M O N P N D F V K D B S N T N E B E S U C A
O N Q I N K V A E F S G R E D U E I Q C S I O P U R I J K M
M H J H R I E E C W L T I W Y E S P U E O N D H N I O J Y P
B T G Y M S T B B G P E E O A B G I N H O F E R D C N S W O
S M O E V B T R A I P W X R P V V R O V K A Z I L A O T P N
X I Y R F Z R D O C E E K Z I L E C E N E R B N E R Q E S A
X T T T I W Z A E G H J R X N O A V P E V C Q E B D U N E D
C R X R B N W L D G L A U I F O R S W U I T N U R I A O P E
X A M O J V D L A Y R Y Y N C O R M T U X I D F A T N S T A
J L R P G S S A S T C E C S C A Y M I Y Y O K Z N I T I A O
F V I H S X V H F A E A E E Y T R P A A F N R L C S E S L R
C A G Y T S T N I E N R R G R S I D C L J D V M H P R Y M T
U L H B E O O X B Y Z O A D M I T O I T S F Z U F T I L I I
W V T R L O O K R I P W D L I Z N O N O F I C R F L O C T C
S E C C E R D D I Z U C A E M A S P L A C A N M L W R A A V
L O O C V E I M L J R R A V R I R Z U E L E Q U N Q M B V A
H O R D A S A V L Z K W S T E N O S I S W H N R S F I D X L
E P O R T T G X A Y I M J B T Y C A Y R Z W Y T S D Y D P V
Q E N O I E O P T D N A E A B T P J Z R K P O K E Z W V X E
B A A B O N N C I H J F F Q V C M A A T B S I P K S W A V E
Y Y R Z N T A W O O E I X P R U G K U V N P Z Z N T I I M Z
J X Y M P F L P N Q X B C A V S K T W E L V E L E A D S E V
```

49

WORD LIST:

ANGIOPLASTY	EPINEPHRINE	PEA	STENOSIS
ANTERIORMI	FIBRILLATION	PERICARDIOCENTESIS	STENOSIS
AORTICVALVE	FIRSTDEGREE	PERICARDITIS	STENT
ATROPINE	HYERTROPHY	PJC	SUPREVENTRICULAR
AVF	HYPERACUTE	POSTERIORMI	SVT
AVL	INFARCTION	PURKINJE	SWAVE
AVNODE	INFERIORMI	PVC	TACHYCARDIA
AVR	JUNCTIONAL	QRS	TAMPONADE
AYSYSTOLE	JVD	QWAVE	TWAVE
BALLOON	LAD	RCA	TWELVELEAD
BRADYCARDIA	LATERALMI	RIGHTCORONARY	VFIB
BUNDLEBRANCH	LCA	RWAVE	VTACH
CIRCUMFLEX	MITRALVALVE	SANODE	WINKEBACH
DIAGONAL	MURMUR	SECONDDEGREE	WPW
EF	NITROGLYCERIN	SEPTALMI	
EFFUSION	NORMALSINUS	STDEPRESSION	
EMBOLECTOMY	PAC	STELEVATION	

You can find the solution for this puzzle at;
https://mywordsearch.com/158461
Password: supernurse

Made in the USA
Coppell, TX
06 October 2021

63531251R00033